The Clean Eating Slow Cooker for Beginners

Tasty and Easy Recipes for You

By David Walton

Sommario

Introduction

We understand you are always seeking less complicated ways to prepare your meals. We additionally recognize you are possibly tired investing long hrs in the cooking area cooking with numerous pans and also pots.
Well, now your search is over! We located the best cooking area tool you can use from now on! We are discussing the Slow cooker! These amazing pots enable you to prepare a few of the very best dishes ever with minimum effort Slow-moving stoves cook your meals much easier as well as a whole lot much healthier! You do not need to be a specialist in the cooking area to prepare some of one of the most delicious, flavorful, textured and abundant meals!
All you need is your Slow stove as well as the ideal ingredients! It will certainly reveal you that you can make some outstanding morning meals, lunch dishes, side recipes, fowl, meat as well as fish dishes.
Lastly yet significantly, this cookbook supplies you some easy and also pleasant desserts.

Slow Cooker Snack Recipes

Tamale Dip

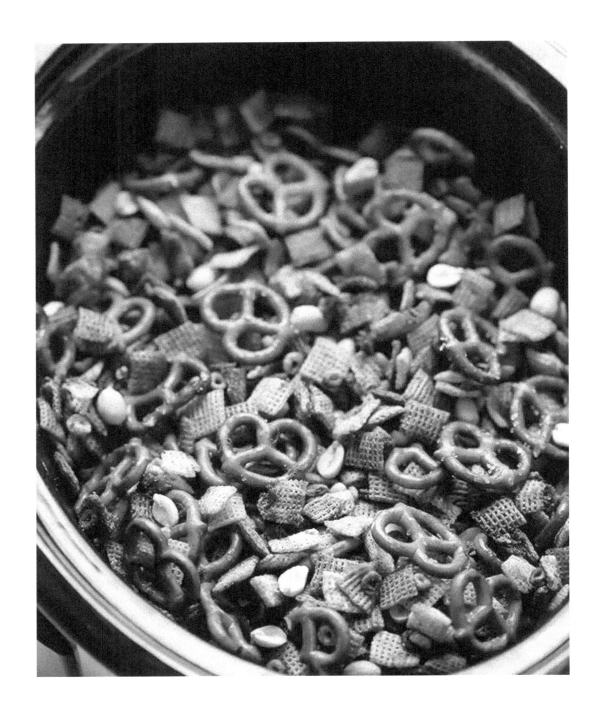

Preparation time: 10 minutes

Cooking time: 2 hours

Servings: 8

Ingredients:

- 1 jalapeno, chopped

- 8 ounces cream cheese, cubed

- ¾ cup cheddar cheese, shredded

- ½ cup Monterey jack cheese, shredded

- 2 garlic cloves, minced

- 15 ounces enchilada sauce

- 1 cup canned corn, drained

- 1 cup rotisserie chicken, shredded

- 1 tablespoon chili powder

- Salt and black pepper to the taste

- 1 tablespoon cilantro, chopped

Directions:

1. In your Slow cooker, mix jalapeno with cream cheese, cheddar cheese, Monterey cheese, garlic, enchilada sauce, corn, chicken, chili powder, salt and pepper, stir, cover and cook on Low for 2 hours.

2. Add cilantro, stir, divide into bowls and serve as a snack.

Nutrition: calories 200, fat 4, fiber 7, carbs 20, protein 4

Spinach Spread

Preparation time: 10 minutes

Cooking time: 2 hours

Servings: 2

Ingredients:

- 4 ounces baby spinach

- 2 tablespoons mayonnaise

- 2 ounces heavy cream

- ½ teaspoon turmeric powder

- A pinch of salt and black pepper

- 1 ounce Swiss cheese, shredded

Directions:

1. In your slow cooker, mix the spinach with the cream, mayo and the other ingredients, toss, put the lid on and cook on Low for 2 hours.

2. Divide into bowls and serve as a party spread.

Nutrition: calories 132, fat 4, fiber 3, carbs 10, protein 4

BBQ Chicken Dip

Preparation time: 10 minutes

Cooking time: 1 hour and 30 minutes

Servings: 10

Ingredients:

- 1 and ½ cups bbq sauce

- 1 small red onion, chopped

- 24 ounces cream cheese, cubed

- 2 cups rotisserie chicken, shredded

- 3 bacon slices, cooked and crumbled

- 1 plum tomato, chopped

- ½ cup cheddar cheese, shredded

- 1 tablespoon green onions, chopped

Directions:

1. In your Slow cooker, mix bbq sauce with onion, cream cheese, rotisserie chicken, bacon, tomato, cheddar and green onions, stir, cover and cook on Low for 1 hour and 30 minutes.

2. Divide into bowls and serve.

Nutrition: calories 251, fat 4, fiber 6, carbs 10, protein 4

Artichoke Dip

Preparation time: 10 minutes

Cooking time: 2 hours

Servings: 2

Ingredients:

- 2 ounces canned artichoke hearts, drained and chopped

- 2 ounces heavy cream

- 2 tablespoons mayonnaise

- ¼ cup mozzarella, shredded

- 2 green onions, chopped

- ½ teaspoon garam masala

- Cooking spray

Directions:

1. Grease your slow cooker with the cooking spray, and mix the artichokes with the cream, mayo and the other ingredients inside.

2. Stir, cover, cook on Low for 2 hours, divide into bowls and serve as a party dip.

Nutrition: calories 100, fat 3, fiber 2, carbs 7, protein 3

Mexican Dip

Preparation time: 10 minutes

Cooking time: 1 hour and 30 minutes

Servings: 10

Ingredients:

- 24 ounces cream cheese, cubed

- 2 cups rotisserie chicken breast, shredded

- 3 ounces canned green chilies, chopped

- 1 and ½ cups Monterey jack cheese, shredded

- 1 and ½ cups salsa Verde

- 1 tablespoon green onions, chopped

Directions:

1. In your Slow cooker, mix cream cheese with chicken, chilies, cheese, salsa Verde and green onions, stir, cover and cook on Low for 1 hour and 30 minutes.

2. Divide into bowls and serve.

Nutrition: calories 222, fat 4, fiber 5, carbs 15, protein 4

Crab Dip

Preparation time: 10 minutes

Cooking time: 1 hour

Servings: 2

Ingredients:

- 2 ounces crabmeat

- 1 tablespoon lime zest, grated

- ½ tablespoon lime juice

- 2 tablespoons mayonnaise

- 2 green onions, chopped

- 2 ounces cream cheese, cubed

- Cooking spray

Directions:

1. Grease your slow cooker with the cooking spray, and mix the crabmeat with the lime zest, juice and the other ingredients inside.

2. Put the lid on, cook on Low for 1 hour, divide into bowls and serve as a party dip.

Nutrition: calories 100, fat 3, fiber 2, carbs 9, protein 4

Tex Mex Dip

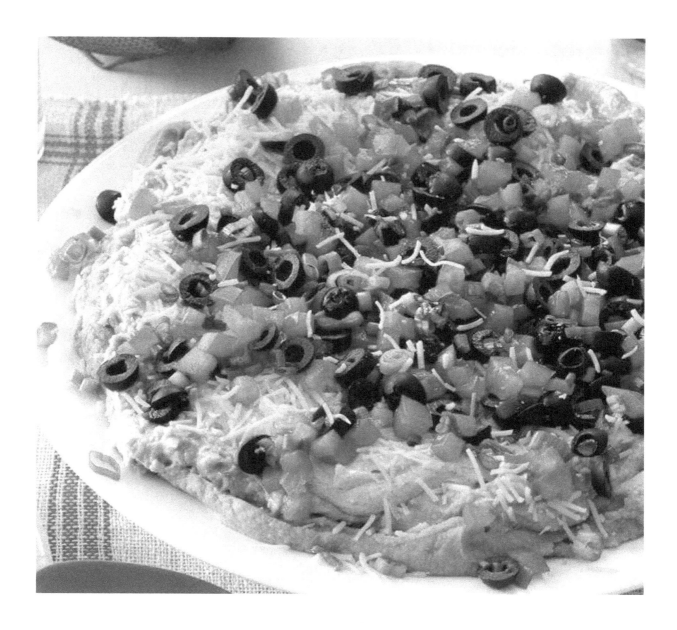

Preparation time: 10 minutes

Cooking time: 1 hour

Servings: 6

Ingredients:

- 15 ounces canned chili con carne

- 1 cup Mexican cheese, shredded

- 1 yellow onion, chopped

- 8 ounces cream cheese, cubed

- ½ cup beer

- A pinch of salt

- 12 ounces macaroni, cooked

- 1 tablespoons cilantro, chopped

Directions:

1. In your Slow cooker, mix chili con carne with cheese, onion, cream cheese, beer and salt, stir, cover and cook on High for 1 hour.

2. Add macaroni and cilantro, stir, divide into bowls and serve.

Nutrition: calories 200, fat 4, fiber 6, carbs 17, protein 5

Lemon Shrimp Dip

Preparation time: 10 minutes

Cooking time: 2 hours

Servings: 2

Ingredients:

- 3 ounces cream cheese, soft

- ½ cup heavy cream

- 1 pound shrimp, peeled, deveined and chopped

- ½ tablespoon balsamic vinegar

- 2 tablespoons mayonnaise

- ½ tablespoon lemon juice

- A pinch of salt and black pepper

- 2 ounces mozzarella, shredded

- 1 tablespoon parsley, chopped

Directions:

1. In your slow cooker, mix the cream cheese with the shrimp, heavy cream and the other ingredients, whisk, put the lid on and cook on Low for 2 hours.

2. Divide into bowls and serve as a dip.

Nutrition: calories 342, fat 4, fiber 3, carbs 7, protein 10

Artichoke Dip

Preparation time: 10 minutes

Cooking time: 2 hours

Servings: 6

Ingredients:

- 10 ounces spinach

- 30 ounces canned artichoke hearts

- 5 ounces boursin

- 1 and ½ cup cheddar cheese, shredded

- ½ cup parmesan, grated

- 2 garlic cloves, minced

- 1 teaspoon red pepper flakes, crushed

- A pinch of salt

Directions:

1. In your Slow cooker mix spinach with artichokes, boursin, cheddar, parmesan, garlic, pepper flakes and salt, stir, cover and cook on High for 1 hour.

2. Stir the dip, cover and cook on Low for 1 more hour.

3. Divide into bowls and serve.

Nutrition: calories 251, fat 6, fiber 8, carbs 16, protein 5

Squash Salsa

Preparation time: 10 minutes

Cooking time: 3 hours

Servings: 2

Ingredients:

- 1 cup butternut squash, peeled and cubed

- 1 cup cherry tomatoes, cubed

- 1 cup avocado, peeled, pitted and cubed

- ½ tablespoon balsamic vinegar

- ½ tablespoon lemon juice

- 1 tablespoon lemon zest, grated

- ¼ cup veggie stock

- 1 tablespoon chives, chopped

- A pinch of rosemary, dried

- A pinch of sage, dried

- A pinch of salt and black pepper

Directions:

1. In your slow cooker, mix the squash with the tomatoes, avocado and the other ingredients, toss, put the lid on and cook on Low for 3 hours.

2. Divide into bowls and serve as a snack.

Nutrition: calories 182, fat 5, fiber 7, carbs 12, protein 5

Taco Dip

Preparation time: 10 minutes

Cooking time: 2 hours and 30 minutes

Servings: 7

Ingredients:

- 1 rotisserie chicken, shredded

- 2 cups pepper jack, cheese, grated

- 15 ounces canned enchilada sauce

- 1 jalapeno, sliced

- 8 ounces cream cheese, soft

- 1 tablespoon taco seasoning

Directions:

1. In your Slow cooker, mix chicken with pepper jack, enchilada sauce, jalapeno, cream and taco seasoning, stir, cover and cook on High for 1 hour.

2. Stir the dip, cover and cook on Low for 1 hour and 30 minutes more.

3. Divide into bowls and serve as a snack.

Nutrition: calories 251, fat 5, fiber 8, carbs 17, protein 5

Beans Spread

Preparation time: 10 minutes

Cooking time: 6 hours

Servings: 2

Ingredients:

- 1 cup canned black beans, drained

- 2 tablespoons tahini paste

- ½ teaspoon balsamic vinegar

- ¼ cup veggie stock

- ½ tablespoon olive oil

Directions:

1. In your slow cooker, mix the beans with the tahini paste and the other ingredients, toss, put the lid on and cook on Low for 6 hours.

2. Transfer to your food processor, blend well, divide into bowls and serve.

Nutrition: calories 221, fat 6, fiber 5, carbs 19, protein 3

Lasagna Dip

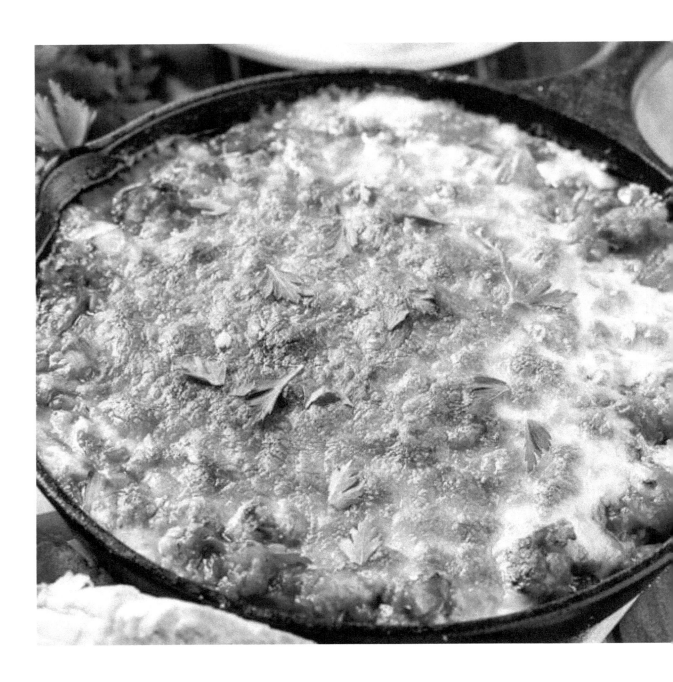

Preparation time: 10 minutes

Cooking time: 1 hour

Servings: 10

Ingredients:

- 8 ounces cream cheese

- ¾ cup parmesan, grated

- 1 and ½ cups ricotta

- ½ teaspoon red pepper flakes, crushed

- 2 garlic cloves, minced

- 3 cups marinara sauce

- 1 and ½ cups mozzarella, shredded

- 1 and ½ teaspoon oregano, chopped

Directions:

1. In your Slow cooker, mix cream cheese with parmesan, ricotta, pepper flakes, garlic, marinara, mozzarella and oregano, stir, cover and cook on High for 1 hour.

2. Stir, divide into bowls and serve as a dip.

Nutrition: calories 231, fat 4, fiber 7, carbs 21, protein 5

Rice Snack Bowls

Preparation time: 10 minutes

Cooking time: 6 hours

Servings: 2

Ingredients:

- ½ cup wild rice

- 1 red onion, sliced

- ½ cup brown rice

- 2 cups veggie stock

- ½ cup baby spinach

- ½ cup cherry tomatoes, halved

- 2 tablespoons pine nuts, toasted

- 1 tablespoon raisins

- 1 tablespoon chives, chopped

- 1 tablespoon dill, chopped

- ½ tablespoon olive oil

- A pinch of salt and black pepper

Directions:

1. In your slow cooker, mix the rice with the onion, stock and the other ingredients, toss, put the lid on and cook on Low for 6 hours.

2. Divide in to bowls and serve as a snack.

Nutrition: calories 301, fat 6, fiber 6, carbs 12, protein 3

Beer and Cheese Dip

Preparation time: 10 minutes

Cooking time: 1 hour

Servings: 10

Ingredients:

- 12 ounces cream cheese
- 6 ounces beer
- 4 cups cheddar cheese, shredded
- 1 tablespoon chives, chopped

Directions:

1. In your Slow cooker, mix cream cheese with beer and cheddar, stir, cover and cook on Low for 1 hour.

2. Stir your dip, add chives, divide into bowls and serve.

Nutrition: calories 212, fat 4, fiber 7, carbs 16, protein 5

Cauliflower Spread

Preparation time: 10 minutes

Cooking time: 7 hours

Servings: 2

Ingredients:

- 1 cup cauliflower florets

- 1 tablespoon mayonnaise

- ½ cup heavy cream

- 1 tablespoon lemon juice

- ½ teaspoon garlic powder

- ¼ teaspoon smoked paprika

- ¼ teaspoon mustard powder

- A pinch of salt and black pepper

Directions:

1. In your slow cooker, combine the cauliflower with the cream, mayonnaise and the other ingredients, toss, put the lid on and cook on Low for 7 hours.

2. Transfer to a blender, pulse well, into bowls and serve as a spread.

Nutrition: calories 152, fat 13.8, fiber 1.5, carbs 6.2, protein 2

Queso Dip

Preparation time: 10 minutes

Cooking time: 1 hour

Servings: 10

Ingredients:

- 16 ounces Velveeta

- 1 cup whole milk

- ½ cup cotija

- 2 jalapenos, chopped

- 2 teaspoons sweet paprika

- 2 garlic cloves, minced

- A pinch of cayenne pepper

- 1 tablespoon cilantro, chopped

Directions:

1. In your Slow cooker, mix Velveeta with milk, cotija, jalapenos, paprika, garlic and cayenne, stir, cover and cook on High for 1 hour.

2. Stir the dip, add cilantro, divide into bowls and serve as a dip.

Nutrition: calories 233, fat 4, fiber 7, carbs 10, protein 4

Mushroom Dip

Preparation time: 10 minutes

Cooking time: 5 hours

Servings: 2

Ingredients:

- 4 ounces white mushrooms, chopped

- 1 eggplant, cubed

- ½ cup heavy cream

- ½ tablespoon tahini paste

- 2 garlic cloves, minced

- A pinch of salt and black pepper

- 1 tablespoon balsamic vinegar

- ½ tablespoon basil, chopped

- ½ tablespoon oregano, chopped

Directions:

1. In your slow cooker, mix the mushrooms with the eggplant, cream and the other ingredients, toss, put the lid on and cook on High for 5 hours.

2. Divide the mushroom mix into bowls and serve as a dip.

Nutrition: calories 261, fat 7, fiber 6, carbs 10, protein 6

Crab Dip

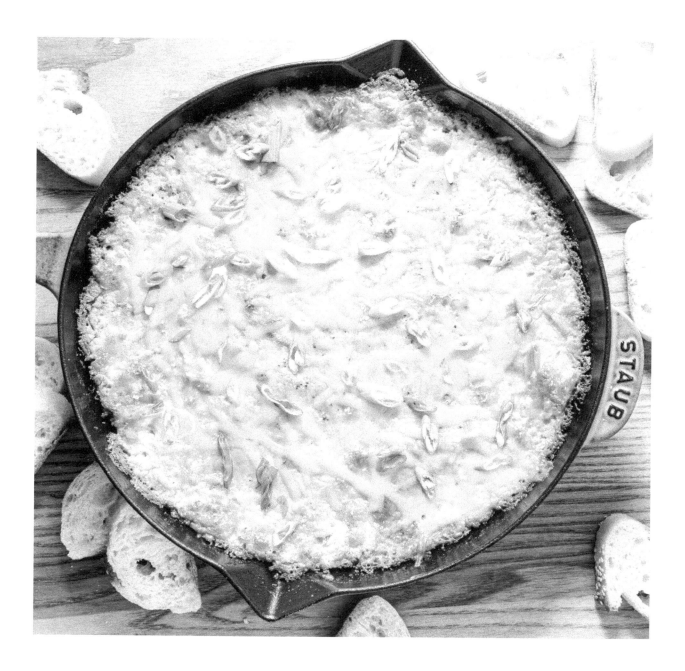

Preparation time: 10 minutes

Cooking time: 2 hours

Servings: 6

Ingredients:

- 12 ounces cream cheese

- ½ cup parmesan, grated

- ½ cup mayonnaise

- ½ cup green onions, chopped

- 2 garlic cloves, minced

- Juice of 1 lemon

- 1 and ½ tablespoon Worcestershire sauce

- 1 and ½ teaspoons old bay seasoning

- 12 ounces crabmeat

Directions:

1. In your Slow cooker, mix cream cheese with parmesan, mayo, green onions, garlic, lemon juice, Worcestershire sauce, old bay seasoning and crabmeat, stir, cover and cook on Low for 2 hours.

2. Divide into bowls and serve as a dip.

Nutrition: calories 200, fat 4, fiber 6, carbs 12, protein 3

Chickpeas Spread

Preparation time: 10 minutes

Cooking time: 8 hours

Servings: 2

Ingredients:

- ½ cup chickpeas, dried
- 1 tablespoons olive oil
- 1 tablespoon lemon juice
- 1 cup veggie stock
- 1 tablespoon tahini
- A pinch of salt and black pepper
- 1 garlic clove, minced
- ½ tablespoon chives, chopped

Directions:

1. In your slow cooker, combine the chickpeas with the stock, salt, pepper and the garlic, stir, put the lid on and cook on Low for 8 hours.

2. Drain chickpeas, transfer them to a blender, add the rest of the ingredients, pulse well, divide into bowls and serve as a party spread.

Nutrition: calories 211, fat 6, fiber 7, carbs 8, protein 4

Corn Dip

Preparation time: 10 minutes

Cooking time: 3 hours

Servings: 12

Ingredients:

- 9 cups corn, rice and wheat cereal

- 1 cup cheerios

- 2 cups pretzels

- 1 cup peanuts

- 6 tablespoons hot, melted butter

- 1 tablespoon salt

- ¼ cup Worcestershire sauce

- 1 teaspoon garlic powder

Directions:

1. In your Slow cooker, mix cereal with cheerios, pretzels, peanuts, butter, salt, Worcestershire sauce and garlic powder, toss well, cover and cook on Low for 3 hours.

2. Divide into bowls and serve as a snack.

Nutrition: calories 182, fat 4, fiber 5, carbs 8, protein 8

Spinach Dip

Preparation time: 10 minutes

Cooking time: 1 hour

Servings: 2

Ingredients:

- 2 tablespoons heavy cream

- ½ cup Greek yogurt

- ½ pound baby spinach

- 2 garlic cloves, minced

- Salt and black pepper to the taste

Directions:

1. In your slow cooker, mix the spinach with the cream and the other ingredients, toss, put the lid on and cook on High for 1 hour.

2. Blend using an immersion blender, divide into bowls and serve as a party dip.

Nutrition: calories 221, fat 5, fiber 7, carbs 12, protein 5

Candied Pecans

Preparation time: 10 minutes

Cooking time: 3 hours

Servings: 4

Ingredients:

- 1 cup white sugar

- 1 and ½ tablespoons cinnamon powder

- ½ cup brown sugar

- 1 egg white, whisked

- 4 cups pecans

- 2 teaspoons vanilla extract

- ¼ cup water

Directions:

1. In a bowl, mix white sugar with cinnamon, brown sugar and vanilla and stir.

2. Dip pecans in egg white, then in sugar mix and put them in your Slow cooker, also add the water, cover and cook on Low for 3 hours.

3. Divide into bowls and serve as a snack.

Nutrition: calories 152, fat 4, fiber 7, carbs 16, protein 6

Dill Potato Salad

Preparation time: 10 minutes

Cooking time: 8 hours

Servings: 2

Ingredients:

- 1 red onion, sliced

- 1 pound gold potatoes, peeled and roughly cubed

- 2 tablespoons balsamic vinegar

- ½ cup heavy cream

- 1 tablespoons mustard

- A pinch of salt and black pepper

- 1 tablespoon dill, chopped

- ½ cup celery, chopped

Directions:

1. In your slow cooker, mix the potatoes with the cream, mustard and the other ingredients, toss, put the lid on and cook on Low for 8 hours.

2. Divide salad into bowls, and serve as an appetizer.

Nutrition: calories 251, fat 6, fiber 7, carbs 8, protein 7

Chicken Bites

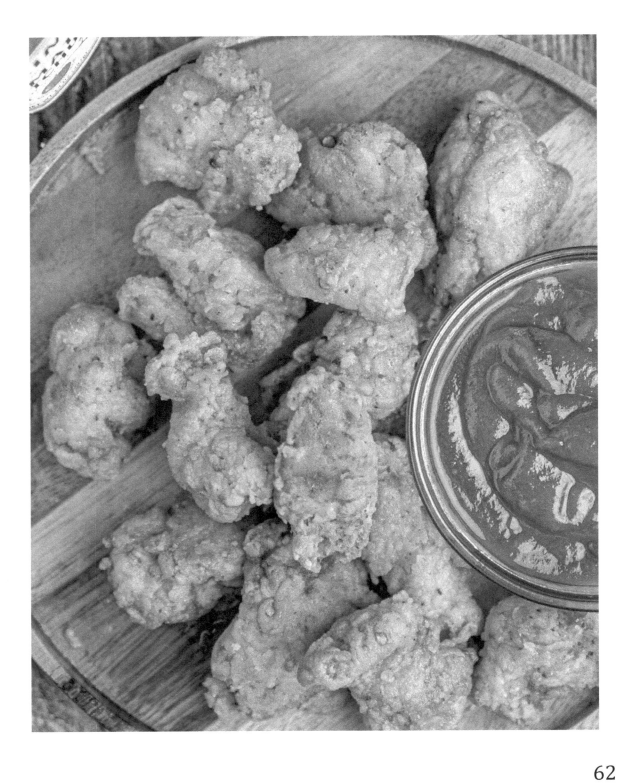

Preparation time: 10 minutes

Cooking time: 7 hours

Servings: 4

Ingredients:

- 1 pound chicken thighs, boneless and skinless

- 1 tablespoon ginger, grated

- 1 yellow onion, sliced

- 1 tablespoon garlic, minced

- 2 teaspoons cumin, ground

- 1 teaspoon cinnamon powder

- 2 tablespoons sweet paprika

- 1 and ½ cups chicken stock

- 2 tablespoons lemon juice

- ½ cup green olives, pitted and roughly chopped

- Salt to the taste

- 3 tablespoons olive oil

- 5 pita breads, cut in quarters and heated in the oven

Directions:

1. Heat up a pan with the olive oil over medium-high heat, add onions, garlic, ginger, salt and pepper, stir and cook for 2 minutes.

2. Add cumin and cinnamon, stir well and take off heat.

3. Put chicken pieces in your Slow cooker, add onions mix, lemon juice, olives and stock, stir, cover and cook on Low for 7 hours.

4. Shred meat, stir the whole mixture again, divide it on pita chips and serve as a snack.

Nutrition: calories 265, fat 7, fiber 6, carbs 14, protein 6

Potato Salsa

Preparation time: 10 minutes

Cooking time: 8 hours

Servings: 6

Ingredients:

- 1 sweet onion, chopped

- ¼ cup white vinegar

- 2 tablespoons mustard

- Salt and black pepper to the taste

- 1 and ½ pounds gold potatoes, cut into medium cubes

- ¼ cup dill, chopped

- 1 cup celery, chopped

- Cooking spray

Directions:

3. Spray your Slow cooker with cooking spray, add onion, vinegar, mustard, salt and pepper and whisk well.

4. Add celery and potatoes, toss them well, cover and cook on Low for 8 hours.

5. Divide salad into small bowls, sprinkle dill on top and serve.

Nutrition: calories 251, fat 6, fiber 7, carbs 12, protein 7

Calamari Rings Bowls

Preparation time: 10 minutes

Cooking time: 6 hours

Servings: 2

Ingredients:

- ½ pound calamari rings

- 1 tablespoon balsamic vinegar

- ½ tablespoon soy sauce

- 1 tablespoon sugar

- 1 cup veggie stock

- ½ teaspoon turmeric powder

- ½ teaspoon sweet paprika

- ½ cup chicken stock

Directions:

1. In your slow cooker, mix the calamari rings with the vinegar, soy sauce and the other ingredients, toss, put the lid on and cook on High for 6 hours.

2. Divide into bowls and serve right away as an appetizer.

Nutrition: calories 230, fat 2, fiber 4, carbs 7, protein 5

Black Bean Salsa Salad

Preparation time: 10 minutes

Cooking time: 4 hours

Servings: 6

Ingredients:

- 1 tablespoon soy sauce

- ½ teaspoon cumin, ground

- 1 cup canned black beans

- 1 cup salsa

- 6 cups romaine lettuce leaves

- ½ cup avocado, peeled, pitted and mashed

Directions:

1. In your slow cooker, mix black beans with salsa, cumin and soy sauce, stir, cover and cook on Low for 4 hours.

2. In a salad bowl, mix lettuce leaves with black beans mix and mashed avocado, toss and serve.

Nutrition: calories 221, fat 4, fiber 7, carbs 12, protein 3

Shrimp Salad

Preparation time: 10 minutes

Cooking time: 2 hours

Servings: 2

Ingredients:

- ½ pound shrimp, peeled and deveined

- 1 green bell pepper, chopped

- ½ cup kalamata olives, pitted and halved

- 4 spring onions, chopped

- 1 red bell pepper, chopped

- ½ cup mild salsa

- 1 tablespoon olive oil

- 1 garlic clove, minced

- ¼ teaspoon oregano, dried

- ¼ teaspoon basil, dried

- Salt and black pepper to the taste

- A pinch of red pepper, crushed

- 1 tablespoon parsley, chopped

Directions:

1. In your slow cooker, mix the shrimp with the peppers and the other ingredients, toss, put the lid on and cook on High for 2 hours.

2. Divide into bowls and serve as an appetizer.

Nutrition: calories 240, fat 2, fiber 5, carbs 7, protein 2

Mushroom Dip

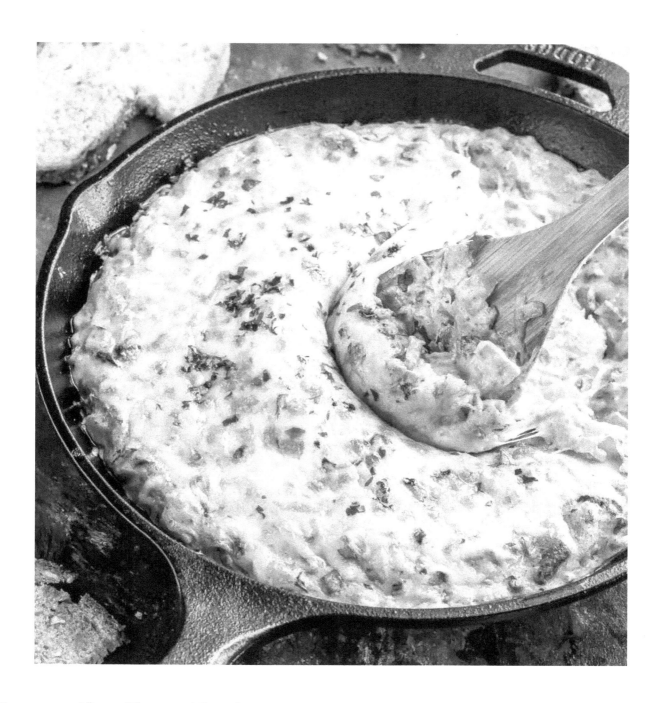

Preparation time: 10 minutes

Cooking time: 4 hours

Servings: 6

Ingredients:

- 2 cups green bell peppers, chopped

- 1 cup yellow onion, chopped

- 3 garlic cloves, minced

- 1 pound mushrooms, chopped

- 28 ounces tomato sauce

- ½ cup goat cheese, crumbled

- Salt and black pepper to the taste

Directions:

3. In your Slow cooker, mix bell peppers with onion, garlic, mushrooms, tomato sauce, cheese, salt and pepper, stir, cover and cook on Low for 4 hours.

4. Divide into bowls and serve.

Nutrition: calories 255, fat 4, fiber 7, carbs 9, protein 3

Chicken Salad

Preparation time: 10 minutes

Cooking time: 6 hours

Servings: 2

Ingredients:

- 2 chicken breasts, skinless, boneless and cubed

- ½ cup mild salsa

- ½ tablespoon olive oil

- 1 red onion, chopped

- ½ cup mushrooms, sliced

- ½ cup kalamata olives, pitted and halved

- ½ cup cherry tomatoes, halved

- 1 chili pepper, chopped

- 2 ounces baby spinach

- 1 teaspoon oregano, chopped

- ½ tablespoon lemon juice

- ½ cup veggie stock

- A pinch of salt and black pepper

Directions:

1. In your slow cooker, mix the chicken with the salsa, oil and the other ingredients except the spinach, toss, put the lid on and cook on High for 5 hours.

2. Add the spinach, cook on High for 1 more hour, divide into bowls and serve as an appetizer.

Nutrition: calories 245, fat 4, fiber 3, carbs 10, protein 6

Beef Meatballs

Preparation time: 10 minutes

Cooking time: 8 hours

Servings: 8

Ingredients:

- 1 and ½ pounds beef, ground

- 1 egg, whisked

- 16 ounces canned tomatoes, crushed

- 14 ounces canned tomato puree

- ¼ cup parsley, chopped

- 2 garlic cloves, minced

- 1 yellow onion, chopped

- Salt and black pepper to the taste

Directions:

1. In a bowl, mix beef with egg, parsley, garlic, black pepper and onion, stir well and shape 16 meatballs.

2. Place them in your slow cooker, add tomato puree and crushed tomatoes on top, cover and cook on Low for 8 hours.

3. Arrange them on a platter and serve.

Nutrition: calories 160, fat 5, fiber 3, carbs 10, protein 7

Apple and Carrot Dip

Preparation time: 10 minutes

Cooking time: 6 hours

Servings: 2

Ingredients:

- 2 cups apples, peeled, cored and chopped

- 1 cup carrots, peeled and grated

- ¼ teaspoon cloves, ground

- ¼ teaspoon ginger powder

- 1 tablespoon lemon juice

- ½ tablespoon lemon zest, grated

- ½ cup coconut cream

- ¼ teaspoon nutmeg, ground

Directions:

1. In your slow cooker, mix the apples with the carrots, cloves and the other ingredients, toss, put the lid on and cook on Low for 6 hours.

2. Bend using an immersion blender, divide into bowls and serve.

Nutrition: calories 212, fat 4, fiber 6, carbs 12, protein 3

Jalapeno Poppers

Preparation time: 10 minutes

Cooking time: 3 hours

Servings: 4

Ingredients:

- ½ pound chorizo, chopped

- 10 jalapenos, tops cut off and deseeded

- 1 small white onion, chopped

- ½ pound beef, ground

- ¼ teaspoon garlic powder

- 1 tablespoon maple syrup

- 1 tablespoon mustard

- 1/3 cup water

Directions:

1. In a bowl, mix beef with chorizo, garlic powder and onion and stir.

2. Stuff your jalapenos with the mix, place them in your Slow cooker, add the water, cover and cook on High for 3 hours.

3. Transfer jalapeno poppers to a lined baking sheet.

4. In a bowl, mix maple syrup with mustard, whisk well, brush poppers with this mix, arrange on a platter and serve.

Nutrition: calories 214, fat 2, fiber 3, carbs 8, protein 3

Sweet Potato Dip

Preparation time: 10 minutes

Cooking time: 4 hours

Servings: 2

Ingredients:

- 2 sweet potatoes, peeled and cubed

- ½ cup coconut cream

- ½ teaspoon turmeric powder

- ½ teaspoon garam masala

- 2 garlic cloves, minced

- ½ cup veggie stock

- 1 cup basil leaves

- 2 tablespoons olive oil

- 1 tablespoon lemon juice

- A pinch of salt and black pepper

Directions:

1. In your slow cooker, mix the sweet potatoes with the cream, turmeric and the other ingredients, toss, put the lid on and cook on High for 4 hours.

2. Blend using an immersion blender, divide into bowls and serve as a party dip.

Nutrition: calories 253, fat 5, fiber 6, carbs 13, protein 4

Pecans Snack

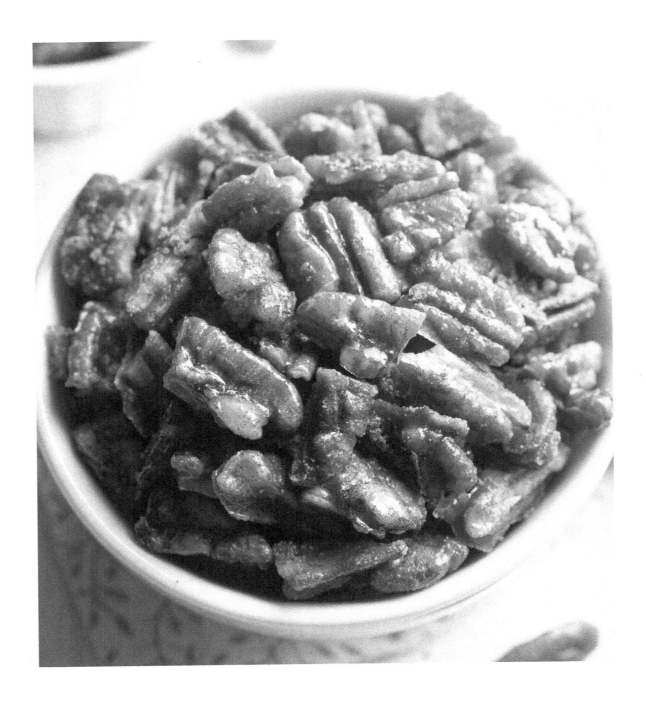

Preparation time: 10 minutes

Cooking time: 2 hours and 15 minutes

Servings: 5

Ingredients:

- 1 pound pecans, halved

- 2 tablespoons olive oil

- 1 teaspoon basil, dried

- 1 tablespoon chili powder

- 1 teaspoon oregano, dried

- ¼ teaspoon garlic powder

- 1 teaspoon thyme, dried

- ½ teaspoon onion powder

- A pinch of cayenne pepper

Directions:

1. In your slow cooker, mix pecans with oil, basil, chili powder, oregano, garlic powder, onion powder, thyme and cayenne and toss to coat.

2. Cover, cook on High for 15 minutes and on Low for 2 hours.

3. Divide into bowls and serve as a snack.

Nutrition: calories 78, fat 3, fiber 2, carbs 9, protein 2

Spinach, Walnuts and Calamari Salad

Preparation time: 10 minutes

Cooking time: 4 hours and 30 minutes

Servings: 2

Ingredients:

- 2 cups baby spinach

- ½ cup walnuts, chopped

- ½ cup mild salsa

- 1 cup calamari rings

- ½ cup kalamata olives, pitted and halved

- ½ teaspoons thyme, chopped

- 2 garlic cloves, minced

- 1 cup tomatoes, cubed

- A pinch of salt and black pepper

- ¼ cup veggie stock

Directions:

3. In your slow cooker, mix the salsa with the calamari rings and the other ingredients except the spinach, toss, put the lid on and cook on High for 4 hours.

4. Add the spinach, toss, put the lid on, cook on High for 30 minutes more, divide into bowls and serve.

Nutrition: calories 160, fat 1, fiber 4, carbs 18, protein 4

Apple Jelly Sausage Snack

Preparation time: 10 minutes

Cooking time: 2 hours

Servings: 15

Ingredients:

- 2 pounds sausages, sliced

- 18 ounces apple jelly

- 9 ounces Dijon mustard

Directions:

1. Place sausage slices in your Slow cooker, add apple jelly and mustard, toss to coat well, cover and cook on Low for 2 hours.

2. Divide into bowls and serve as a snack.

Nutrition: calories 200, fat 3, fiber 1, carbs 9, protein 10

Chicken Meatballs

Preparation time: 10 minutes

Cooking time: 7 hours

Servings: 2

Ingredients:

- A pinch of red pepper flakes, crushed

- ½ pound chicken breast, skinless, boneless, ground

- 1 egg, whisked

- ½ cup salsa Verde

- 1 teaspoon oregano, dried

- ½ teaspoon chili powder

- ½ teaspoon rosemary, dried

- 1 tablespoon parsley, chopped

- A pinch of salt and black pepper

Directions:

1. In a bowl, mix the chicken with the egg and the other ingredients except the salsa, stir well and shape medium meatballs out of this mix.

2. Put the meatballs in the slow cooker, add the salsa Verde, toss gently, put the lid on and cook on Low for 7 hours.

3. Arrange the meatballs on a platter and serve.

Nutrition: calories 201, fat 4, fiber 5, carbs 8, protein 2

Eggplant Dip

Preparation time: 10 minutes

Cooking time: 4 hours and 10 minutes

Servings: 4

Ingredients:

- 1 eggplant

- 1 zucchini, chopped

- 2 tablespoons olive oil

- 2 tablespoons balsamic vinegar

- 1 tablespoon parsley, chopped

- 1 yellow onion, chopped

- 1 celery stick, chopped

- 1 tomato, chopped

- 2 tablespoons tomato paste

- 1 and ½ teaspoons garlic, minced

- A pinch of sea salt

- Black pepper to the taste

Directions:

1. Brush eggplant with the oil, place on preheated grill and cook over medium-high heat for 5 minutes on each side.

2. Leave aside to cool down, chop it and put in your Slow cooker.

3. Also add, zucchini, vinegar, onion, celery, tomato, parsley, tomato paste, garlic, salt and pepper and stir everything.

4. Cover and cook on High for 4 hours.

5. Stir your spread again very well, divide into bowls and serve.

Nutrition: calories 110, fat 1, fiber 2, carbs 7, protein 5

Cinnamon Pecans Snack

Preparation time: 10 minutes

Cooking time: 3 hours

Servings: 2

Ingredients:

- ½ tablespoon cinnamon powder

- ¼ cup water

- ½ tablespoon avocado oil

- ½ teaspoon chili powder

- 2 cups pecans

Directions:

1. In your slow cooker, mix the pecans with the cinnamon and the other ingredients, toss, put the lid on and cook on Low for 3 hours.

2. Divide the pecans into bowls and serve as a snack.

Nutrition: calories 172, fat 3, fiber 5, carbs 8, protein 2

Lemon Peel Snack

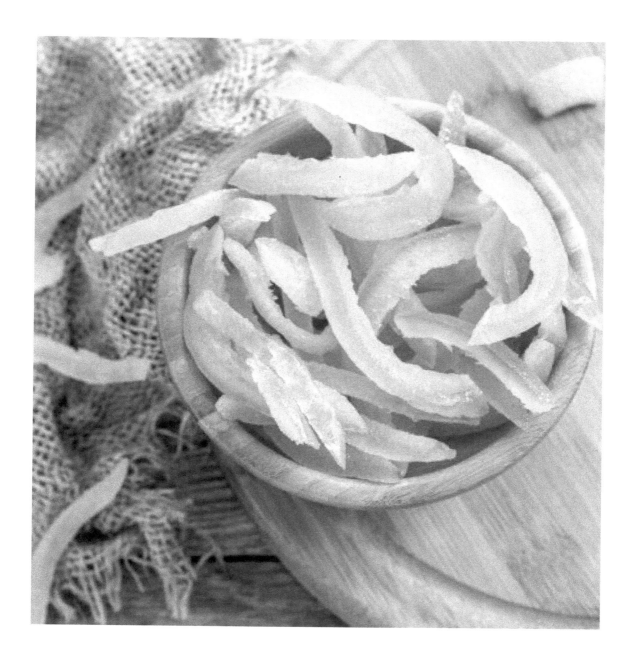

Preparation time: 20 minutes

Cooking time: 4 hours

Servings: 80 pieces

Ingredients:

- 5 big lemons, sliced halves, pulp removed and peel cut into strips
- 2 and ¼ cups white sugar
- 5 cups water

Directions:

1. Put strips in your instant slow cooker, add water and sugar, stir cover and cook on Low for 4 hours.

2. Drain lemon peel and keep in jars until serving.

Nutrition: calories 7, fat 1, fiber 1, carbs 2, protein 1

Cajun Almonds and Shrimp Bowls

Preparation time: 10 minutes

Cooking time: 2 hours

Servings: 2

Ingredients:

- 1 cup almonds

- 1 pound shrimp, peeled and deveined

- ½ cup kalamata olives, pitted and halved

- ½ cup black olives, pitted and halved

- ½ cup mild salsa

- ½ tablespoon Cajun seasoning

Directions:

1. In your slow cooker, mix the shrimp with the almonds, olives and the other ingredients, toss, put the lid on and cook on High for 2 hours.

2. Divide between small plates and serve as an appetizer.

Nutrition: calories 100, fat 2, fiber 3, carbs 7, protein 3

Fava Bean Dip

Preparation time: 10 minutes

Cooking time: 5 hours

Servings: 6

Ingredients:

- 1 pound fava bean, rinsed

- 1 cup yellow onion, chopped

- 4 and ½ cups water

- 1 bay leaf

- ¼ cup olive oil

- 1 garlic clove, minced

- 2 tablespoons lemon juice

- Salt to the taste

Directions:

1. Put fava beans in your Slow cooker, add 4 cups water, salt and bay leaf, cover and cook on Low for 3 hours.

2. Drain beans, discard bay leaf, return beans to the slow cooker, add ½ cup water, garlic and onion, stir, cover and cook on Low for 2 more hours.

3. Transfer beans mix to your food processor, add olive oil and lemon juice and blend well.

4. Divide into bowls and serve cold.

Nutrition: calories 300, fat 3, fiber 1, carbs 20, protein 6

Broccoli Dip

Preparation time: 10 minutes

Cooking time: 2 hours

Servings: 2

Ingredients:

- 1 green chili pepper, minced

- 2 tablespoons heavy cream

- 1 cup broccoli florets

- 1 tablespoon mayonnaise

- 2 tablespoons cream cheese, cubed

- A pinch of salt and black pepper

- 1 tablespoon chives, chopped

Directions:

1. In your slow cooker, mix the broccoli with the chili pepper, mayo and the other ingredients, toss, put the lid on and cook on Low for 2 hours.

2. Blend using an immersion blender, divide into bowls and serve as a party dip.

Nutrition: calories 202, fat 3, fiber 3, carbs 7, protein 6

Tamales

Preparation time: 10 minutes

Cooking time: 8 hours and 30 minutes

Servings: 24

Ingredients:

- 8 ounces dried corn husks, soaked for 1 day and drained

- 4 cups water

- 3 pounds pork shoulder, boneless and chopped

- 1 yellow onion, chopped

- 2 garlic cloves, crushed

- 1 tablespoon chipotle chili powder

- 2 tablespoons chili powder

- Salt and black pepper to the taste

- 1 teaspoon cumin, ground

- 4 cups masa harina

- ¼ cup corn oil

- ¼ cup shortening

- 1 teaspoon baking powder

Directions:

1. In your Slow cooker, mix 2 cups water with salt, pepper, onion, garlic, chipotle powder, chili powder, cumin and pork, stir, cover the slow cooker and cook on Low for 7 hours.

2. Transfer meat to a cutting board, shred it with2 forks, add to a bowl, mix with 1 tablespoon of cooking liquid, more salt and pepper, stir and leave aside.

3. In another bowl, mix masa harina with salt, pepper, baking powder, shortening and oil and stir using a mixer.

4. Add cooking liquid from the instant slow cooker and blend again well.

5. Unfold corn husks, place them on a work surface, add ¼ cup masa mix near the top of the husk, press into a square and leaves 2 inches at the bottom.

6. Add 1 tablespoon pork mix in the center of the masa, wrap the husk around the dough, place all of them in your Slow cooker, add the rest of the water, cover and cook on High for 1 hour and 30 minutes.

7. Arrange tamales on a platter and serve.

Nutrition: calories 162, fat 4, fiber 3, carbs 10, protein 5

Walnuts Bowls

Preparation time: 10 minutes

Cooking time: 2 hours

Servings: 2

Ingredients:

- Cooking spray

- 1 cup walnuts, chopped

- 2 tablespoons balsamic vinegar

- 1 tablespoon smoked paprika

- ½ tablespoon lemon zest, grated

- ½ tablespoons olive oil

- 1 teaspoon rosemary, dried

Directions:

1. Grease your slow cooker with the cooking spray, add walnuts and the other ingredients inside, toss, put the lid on and cook on Low for 2 hours.

2. Divide into bowls and serve them as a snack.

Nutrition: calories 100, fat 2, fiber 2, carbs 3, protein 2

Tostadas

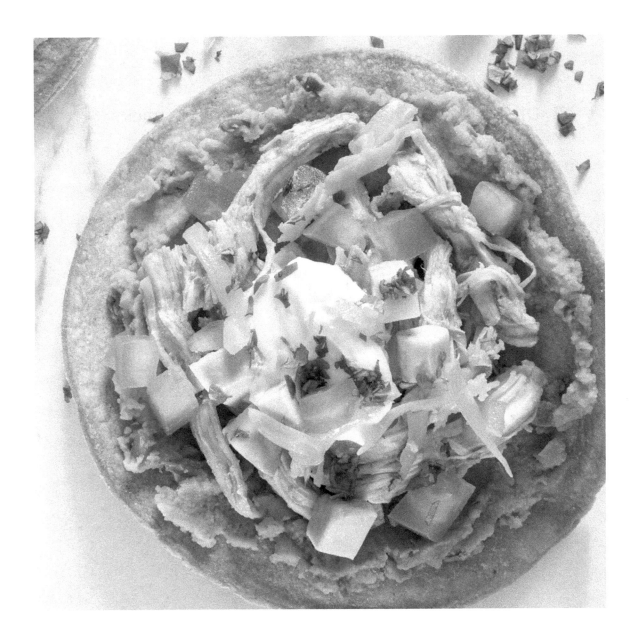

Preparation time: 10 minutes

Cooking time: 4 hours

Servings: 4

Ingredients:

- 4 pounds pork shoulder, boneless and cubed

- Salt and black pepper to the taste

- 2 cups coca cola

- 1/3 cup brown sugar

- ½ cup hot sauce

- 2 teaspoons chili powder

- 2 tablespoons tomato paste

- ¼ teaspoon cumin, ground

- 1 cup enchilada sauce

- Corn tortillas, toasted for a few minutes in the oven

- Mexican cheese, shredded for serving

- 4 shredded lettuce leaves, for serving

- Salsa

- Guacamole for serving

Directions:

1. In your Slow cooker, mix 1 cup coke with hot sauce, salsa, sugar, tomato paste, chili powder, cumin and pork, stir, cover and cook on Low for 4 hours.

2. Drain juice from the slow cooker, transfer meat to a cutting board, shred it, return it to slow cooker, add the rest of the coke and enchilada sauce and stir.

3. Place tortillas on a working surface, divide pork mix, lettuce leaves, Mexican cheese and guacamole and serve as a snack.

Nutrition: calories 162, fat 3, fiber 6, carbs 12, protein 5

Cauliflower Bites

Preparation time: 10 minutes

Cooking time: 4 hours

Servings: 2

Ingredients:

- 2 cups cauliflower florets

- 1 tablespoon Italian seasoning

- 1 tablespoon sweet paprika

- 2 tablespoons tomato sauce

- 1 teaspoon sweet paprika

- 1 tablespoon olive oil

- ¼ cup veggie stock

Directions:

1. In your slow cooker, mix the cauliflower florets with the Italian seasoning and the other ingredients, toss, put the lid on and cook on Low for 4 hours.

2. Divide into bowls and serve as a snack.

Nutrition: calories 251, fat 4, fiber 6, carbs 7, protein 3

Mussels Salad

Preparation time: 10 minutes

Cooking time: 1 hour

Servings: 4

Ingredients:

- 2 pounds mussels, cleaned and scrubbed

- 1 radicchio, cut into thin strips

- 1 white onion, chopped

- 1 pound baby spinach

- ½ cup dry white wine

- 1 garlic clove, crushed

- ½ cup water

- A drizzle of olive oil

Directions:

1. Divide baby spinach and radicchio in salad bowls and leave aside for now.

2. In your Slow cooker, mix mussels with onion, wine, garlic, water and oil, toss, cover and cook on High for 1 hour.

3. Divide mussels on top of spinach and radicchio, add cooking liquid all over and serve.

Nutrition: calories 59, fat 4, fiber 1, carbs 1, protein 1

Conclusion

Did you delight in trying these brand-new as well as scrumptious dishes?

unfortunately we have actually come to the end of this vegan recipe book, I really hope it has been to your liking. to enhance your health we would like to suggest you to integrate physical activity and also a dynamic lifestyle in addition to adhere to these fantastic recipes, so regarding emphasize the enhancements. we will be back soon with various other significantly appealing vegan dishes, a big hug, see you soon.

CPSIA information can be obtained
at www.ICGtesting.com
Printed in the USA
BVHW060019040521
606340BV00002B/232

9 781667 134925